HOW YOGA HARMS

A Love Letter To Understanding Yoga From A Christian Perspective

Michal Russo

CONTENTS

Title Page

Copyright

Namaste   4

My Testimony   7

Yoga is Holy.   13

Everything in Sanskrit is Sacred.   15

The Problem With Christian Yoga   24

What's Really Wrong With Just Doing The Poses?   26

Bibliography   30

About The Author   34

Books By This Author   36

Dear Brothers and Sisters In Christ,

I am writing this as a love letter of sorts, out of desperation to unveil a harmful deception that is operating in the world, and in the body of Christ at these times. I won't waste time beating around the bush. Simply put, yoga is not for Christians. If that statement makes you wince and shrug your shoulders and say, "Now they've gone too far"... I can assure you, I felt that way once too. In fact, I battled with myself over this for more than a decade, ignoring the convictions by the Holy Spirit that tugged at my heart strings and I turned my eyes away from all of the red flags that would pop up along the way. I had convictions about certain philosophies, healing arts, references to sexuality and other advice given to teachers and students of yoga along my journey, but I chose to rationalize the obvious answers into non-truths, which made me feel more comfortable about continuing my yoga practice. I did not allow myself to seek Christ's view, or to truly know the answers from a biblical perspective. After a perilous adventure into becoming a "yogini" with the fullness of my being, and engaging in New Age and counterfeit Christ practices alongside it, I wound up in a world full of utter chaos, destruction,and downright evil that was wreaking havoc in every aspect of my life. I finally turned my face back to the Lord in complete surrender through repentance, and denounced those old ways that I had come to idolize and worship above Him. So thus, the creation of this guide, which is a collection of topics that many believers have come to question as yoga has skyrocketed into mainstream society, and into many Christian's lives.

I nonchalantly practiced yoga for over a decade before traveling overseas to attend a yogashala institute and receive my teacher's certificate. Upon my return back to the United States, I attained a yoga alliance membership and began teaching Hatha Vinyasa at hot yoga studios, fitness centers, and to the US Army. I still refused to acknowledge that what I was practicing was anything spiritual, even though deep down, because of my studies and the research of Hindu texts/philosophy that were required to obtain my certifications, I knew it was more than "just exercise".

As believers, we have welcomed The Holy Spirit into our lives. As we share life with Him, He heeds us with warning signs that we feel internally, or physically even see and hear externally. Since I was born into a Christian household, I knew this all too well. Yet, I persisted to disagree with the others around me who tried to warn me, and I disagreed with my own spirit that chose to ignore the Holy Spirit's convictions. A lot of it had to do with the fact that I was rebelling against the institution of religion itself. I didn't want to live a life of judgment and condemnation, and I had the entirely wrong idea of what a relationship with Christ truly looked and felt like.

The world is really great at making those of us who follow God and call out evil for evil, and good for good, as those who "judge". It was easy to fall into the lure of New Age and yogic philosophies where "everything in the universe is divine". I was ready to run into the seemingly all accepting and tolerant arms of the universe where "unity is love and light". In actuality, we've already been warned about this in the Book of 2 Corinthians 11:14, that it is Satan himself masking as the angel of light. Yoga and the ancillary practices that it promotes and leads many of its students and teachers to are doused in deceptive false light. It looks good, it even feels good, and it sounds good. It is promoted and reiterated as harmless by many, but it is, at its core, an anti-christ spiritual experience that will taint your entire being: body, soul, and spirit.

NAMASTE

You are probably familiar with this term that is so casually thrown around in yoga classes, placed on t-shirts and mugs, and in memes. But, do you know what it actually means, and how it is *supposed* to be used? "Namaste" is Sanskrit for "I bow to you", and it beckons the Hindu belief that there is a bit of God in everyone. Thus, the bow is considered to say "the divine in me recognizes and honors the divine in you"[1]. When asked to explain this as a yoga teacher, I used to water it down as many other teachers often do in order to keep the class comfortable when explaining spiritual facets of yogic terms, and I'd say "the light in me honors the light in you". Most people would shrug and say, "well that sounds harmless enough" and go along with it while taking a bow. In fact, to misuse this term is highly offensive, like the memes you may have seen online that say things like "nama'slay the day" or "nama'stay in bed in my pj's". Why would this be so offensive? Well, because the term is considered by many in the East to be one used with reverence and respect, for it is believed to be "extremely powerful and spiritually resonant"[2]. The use and misuse of this common term is an excellent glimpse into the way we can view each and every aspect of yoga, as well as its individual aspects. It *is* a very spiritual practice to those who traditionally use it, it is done with respect to spirituality to those who created it, and to hundreds of millions who still practice it in the East as it was intended. Yoga, for them, is done out of honor and reverence, and not something to be treated like a casual saturday stretching exercise, just like "Namaste" is not a casual way of saying "alright class is over, see ya later", or even worse, made into a comical meme.

If they find these things offensive, why aren't we willing to see their reluctance to relinquish the sacred nature of yoga and its aspects as an apparent discord to what we've been taught here in the West? Why aren't we willing to see that doing something so seemingly harmless as bowing to our yoga teacher and the rest of the class is completely offensive to The Lord? He made it very clear in His commandments to us that He doesn't take an act like bowing to any other person, thing, or god lightly. God says "You shall not bow down to them or worship them; for I, the LORD your God, am a jealous God, punishing the children for the sin of the parents to the third and fourth generation of those who hate me" (Exodus 20:5, NIV). If we are bowing in yoga, if others are offended by our misuse of their sacred terms, then why are we so eager to argue that it is all just simply breathing and stretching? Why do we think that somehow what we decide in our own minds and hearts changes the root and essence of an ancient sacred practice, and if that is your intention then you are successfully separating the spiritual stuff from it?

As someone who tried to do this "separation of powers" for over a decade, I beg to differ, and my heart pleads that you will consider the following numerous points to arrive at your own spiritual posture aligned with Christ. You see, I thought I had a "good excuse" because I was burned. I had church hurt, family hurt, and overall people hurt, so I took what looked like the lighter route of walking away from the church and towards "spirituality". If you asked me if I was still a Christian, I would have said yes, because I never stopped loving Jesus, but I became what some might call a really bad friend to Him. I became lukewarm. I just quit talking to Him (mostly), I ignored Him when He called, and I definitely was no longer walking with Him. Sure, I'd turn up at the occasional Sunday morning service, but mostly out of reverence to wanting to raise my child up right, albeit I wasn't doing it right for myself at the time.

MY TESTIMONY

Eventually, and pretty publicly I might add, it all led me into a complete crash and burn scenario that left me utterly shattered and broken. Lo and behold, the problems I had gotten myself into, I had no idea how to get myself out of, and no force in "the universe", or special crystal, or balanced chakra could be relied on to pull me up and out of it either.

I promise to make this story of my personal journey as brief as possible. After all, we do have several topics on yoga to explore both intellectually and spiritually in the coming pages. However, I think my testimony is most relevant, and must be shared before I continue on about "How Yoga Harms", because I myself ignored the Holy Spirit and others who tried to warn me since they weren't yoga teachers. Most of the people that sent me articles about how dangerous the underlying yogic spirits are and how it would open doors to New Age and other spirituality practices had never even gone to a yoga class. I simply wrote them off as "kooky christians" who were judging me and others. In fact, their convictions are what actually helped push me farther away from Christ rather than towards

Him. So, let's quickly jump into the good stuff, well, really it's the bad stuff that led me to the "good stuff" (Jesus Christ).

My journey into yoga did eventually open doors that led me into the New Age. It did not happen all at once, and to be honest, now that I look back I don't know how I ever let myself slide down such a slippery slope. However, when I hit rock bottom, I finally began to recognize certain things I'd begun to do as probably not aligned with Christianity. Again, none of this happened quickly or suddenly. I certainly didn't see where I would end up from the start when I was just a highschool girl trying to be cool and fit in by doing the latest "trendy workout" called "yoga" in Miami, Florida back in 2003. I certainly didn't have the intention of doing anything bad at all. In fact I thought it was all "good", and like most slippery slopes are, I never saw the next slip coming until the snowball effect happened and a simple workout led me to believing and practicing an array of other things, and what is now very clearly pagan worship and idolatry to me.

These started out really harmless, with things that yogis and even society use as supplements to well-being. Things like using crystals to alter my energy and sound vibrations. I was basically assigning them values and virtues like stress reducing powers, focus powers, and even healing powers. I used specific ones for specific ailments and really believed that they were going to do things for me like increase my spiritual awareness, enhance creativity, help me avoid negative emotions from my past, bring me abundance, and offer protection and grounding. This is a pretty common New Age practice at this point in the world, and it's even become fashionable to buy bracelets and necklaces with different crystals on them to help harness and attract specific positive energies, or even deflect negative energies. I started incorporating crystals into my yoga classes, using them to direct the theme and intention of each class, like rose quartz for heart healing (emotional and physical) and then we would practice heart opening poses to correspond like Ardvha Purvattanasan, or "reverse table" in English. See that's another thing, every yoga pose has a Sanskrit name, and every single pose is intentional, no matter how harmless the name translates to, like "fish pose" (Matsyasana), or "camel pose" (Ustrasana). You may not be worshiping a fish or a camel by doing them, but they are also intentionally used and designed to open the heart in Hindu philosophy. We will dive more into the sacred nature of Sanskrit and poses in just a moment, but first back to my slippery slope story, so you can see how I arrived where I ended up. It is my honest hope and prayer that my story will spare you from making the same mistakes I did, by trying to self-rationalize my own way out.

After I had some experience using crystals, I learned that specific ones correspond not just to energies, but energy wheels in my body called "chakras". That's why poses like "heart openers" were believed to be spiritually and physically connected, because they corresponded to the "heart chakra". So, I studied those next, and I began to incorporate chakra cleansing and balancing workshops into my yoga teaching practice. "Chakra" is a Sanskrit word that means "wheel", and in my workshops we would work from the root chakra at the base of the tailbone all the way up to the crown chakra on the top of our heads. People would come to these workshops for healing. If a chakra was blocked, the belief is that this could be the reason they were experiencing things like: Anxiety, instability, low self esteem, lack of love and compassion, disconnection from gut instincts and intuitions, and even spiritual connection to themselves, others, and "the universe". We would flow through tuning yoga poses to unblock any that might be unbalanced, utilize the corresponding crystals to the chakra and energy blockage, and we did all of this truly believing that by doing so we were improving the inner self on a physical and spiritual level. I won't go into much more detail here, but it is an ancient practice, and therefore I thought it must be safe, I just ignored the fact that it was an ancient Hindu practice.

In fact, I was recently shocked to find out that one of the institutions that aligns itself as "christian yoga", or "holy yoga", actually includes the teaching of chakras in their course modules. I get it, I was once there too as a "christian yogi" who thought it was harmless and simply supplemental to my belief in Christ. I mean, I couldn't possibly be replacing Christ by spending time focusing so much on these mystical inner powerhouse wheels, and using things like crystals, guided meditations, Sanskrit chants (mantras) and mudras (a symbolic hand gesture intentionally used to conjure up healing power in Hinduism, Buddhism and Jainisim), right?!

So many people use the word "mantra" today and don't even recognize that it is a Sanskrit word which literally means "mind" (man) "train" (tra). By reciting certain words, or more traditionally sounds, you are "activating energies". For example, the *bija mantra* or seed sound RAM (pronounced "rum") is said to induce confidence and focus by activating the energy center associated with the power of the sun, behind the navel, which is known as the *manipura chakra.*[3]

Maybe you're thinking: "Okay, I have never dabbled with chanting mantras, or using crystals, or any of this other stuff in my yoga practice. I just simply breathed and stretched through poses." I hear you, and I was just like you in the beginning too. Maybe you even partake in what some call "Christian Yoga", and think that you are able to separate the original yoga and its intended spirituality by replacing it with Christ. I'm going to share in the rest of this book exactly why that can not be done, I'm going to use ancient texts that were written by the founders of Yoga, the people that created it, and shed light on what every bit of the practice truly means. It is far deeper than "stretching and breathing", I can assure you. That is why it is ascribed as a "body, mind, and soul" practice after all.

I am going to explain why yoga, in its very root and essence, is a spiritual practice which can not be replaced or disconnected from its original and intended purpose. I will do so with all of the grace and compassion of Christ that I have prayed for to relay this important message, so that more of His children do not fall for the same deceptive lies that I did. All of this ultimately led me, to put it nicely, much farther away from Christ, and into counterfeit Christ practices, pagan worship, and idolatry.

YOGA IS HOLY.

The root and essence of yoga is sacred and holy. That is a historical fact based on the mystic sages that developed it, how they defined it, why they practiced it, and what they were using it for. I will go into deep historical and philosophical detail, referencing all sorts of ancient and modern texts by yogic experts and founders, so you don't have to just take my word for it. I know myself ten years ago certainly wouldn't have. Of course, as I practiced and taught yoga, I was reluctant to admit all of this. Afterall, I was doing all of these things with good intentions, and that is the appeal of yoga, isn't it? We do it to seek inner balance, health, peace, and to reduce stress and anxiety. So, I really didn't want to believe that the poses and sequences of poses, let alone the Sanskrit chanting and mudras, were all considered spiritually sacred by others, and an offering to roughly 330 million other gods than my own. In fact, at the end, I was more intentional about showing up to my three or more classes a day to teach at the yoga studio than I was about making it to church on a Sunday. I fully believed this was where my help, my peace, my joy and my "fullness" was flowing from. I was also ashamed to admit that the minute I left the studio, the reality of my shattering "real life" would come crashing down on me hard. Eventually, I was not even seeking The One who promises all of this goodness in the Fruits of the Spirit (love, joy, peace, patience, kindness, goodness, faithfulness, gentleness, and self control) if only I had trusted in Him, who is fully holy, instead of yoga.

Let's begin there, by explaining Sanskrit, the language used in every word of the practice of "yoga".

EVERYTHING IN SANSKRIT IS SACRED.

Sanskrit is a liturgical language, and therefore sacred. It is mainly only written and read, rarely spoken, and primarily used for religious reasons by people who otherwise speak another language in their everyday lives. If you were to travel out to India and the surrounding regions where yoga originated, you would not find anyone natively speaking Sanskrit today. For us Christians, this would be akin to Ancient Hebrew or even Aramaic, the language used by the Apostles, the early Jewish converts, and even by Our Lord.[4] These languages are now considered "dead" and only live in ancient texts, like the Dead Sea Scrolls. Thankfully, scholars have worked over thousands of years to translate them for us into our modern languages so we can understand them, but just imagine if they had not. Imagine if you had to learn those ancient languages just to read the Bible, that is what those who learn to read and speak Sanskrit have to do to understand the Vedas (the sacred texts where yoga is first mentioned). We can also look to the Greek Orthodox church who still uses Koine Greek, as seen in the Pauline Epistles and much of the New Testament, but never spoken or heard in modern day Greece today. The Roman Catholic church is another example where we can gain further insight and analogy. They have ascribed to using Latin as their liturgical language, and they make it very clear that the use of this language is sacred and holy. In fact, to replace it with the vernacular during holy rites and sacraments would be a grave and serious offense. Pope Pius x, the former head of the Catholic Church reaffirmed this in his motu proprio *Tr Le Sollecitudini* (1903), that "the language proper to the

Roman Church is Latin and hence it is forbidden to sing anything whatsoever in the vernacular in solemn liturgical functions- more more to sing in the vernacular the variable or common parts of the Mass and Office".[5] We, however, have no problem throwing around the sacred Sanskrit words like "yoga", "asana", "pranayama" and so on. I will get into detail of what each of these common yogic terms mean in a moment, but first I think we need to solidify the idea that, when recognized as holy, it must now seem odd that we often even refer to things such as leggings, i.e. "yoga pants" as "sacred yoking to the Divine [Supreme Spirit] pants". It's almost silly sounding when we properly translate it that way, isn't it? Yet, that is the true meaning and definition of the word!

Yoga is Sanskrit for "yoke".

Now I will go into the very meaning of the common words you may hear and even use without otherwise knowing their true definitions, and we will start at the very beginning with the word "yoga". "Yoga" is a Sanskrit word that means "to yoke". It comes from the Sanskrit root words "yuj" and "yujir" and these actually mean "to connect" and "to yoke".

Let's break that down for a second, because it is most important that we understand this as it is directly relevant to the root and essence of yoga, a sacred one that can not be broken no matter what else we may call it or try to change it to in our minds and hearts. It is what it is, and it is a practice that means to "yoke" or "connect" and it's not even an English word, it is a language that was developed as sacred in Hinduism and Hinduism philosophy during the Vedic period, as well as the historical texts of Buddhism and Jainism.

We have already looked at how other religions use liturgical languages, so we can now understand that Sanskrit is sacred, and that it is a language that was originally used to communicate with the Hindu celestial gods. The Vedic [mystical] priests developed the practice of "yoga" to connect and yoke with their Divine. Just to be clear, this Divine with a capital "D" is not our Divine, which is God (YHWH). Every word traditionally used during yoga is also Sanskrit, like "asana" which means "pose", "pranayama" which is breathing exercises, and many more that we will soon get into, but for the sake of understanding this most fundamental, I want to make clear that the language and name of "Yoga" is sacred and has deeply spiritual ancient roots.

"The Father of Yoga"[6] is considered by many to be a man named Patanjali. He was a Hindu mystic, philosopher, and Author of "The Yoga Sutras". Many in the Hindu tradition consider Patanjali to be more than a man, but a divine figure as he authored sacred Sanskrit texts on both yoga and ayurveda. He is also listed as one of 26 mythical divine serpents in a number of Puranas, which are more sacred Hindu texts written by a sage named Veda Vyasa.[7] Patanjali's Yoga Sutras is a required reading for most yoga teachers (I had to read a version of it for my certification and know most other yoga institutes require it too). In his writings, Patanjali outlines some key verses that we will look at as translated into English from Sanskrit by Swami Vivekananda. It is regarded as one of the most influential commentaries on modern yoga.[8]

In verse 1.2 of Patanjali's Yoga Sutras, we see the Sanskrit "Yogashchittavrittinirodhah", which means "Yoga is restraining the mind-stuff (Chitta) from taking various forms (Vrttis)" according to Swami Vivekananda's translation.[9] He goes into further detail by stating, "Chitta manifests itself in all these different forms - scattering, darkening, weakening, and concentrating"[10], and he gives attribute to angels and demons possessing this mind-stuff when he notes that these are the "four states in which the mind-stuff manifests itself."[11] According to Swami Vivekananda there is "first a scattered form, activity" with a "tendency to manifest in the form of pleasure or of pain"[12]. There is a darker form of Chitta he refers to as " the dull form" and it "is darkness, the only tendency of which is to injure others."[13] He attributes, "the first form as natural to the Devas, the angels, and the second is the demoniacal form."[14] To know that when one partakes in yoga they are dabbling with forces that can even be attributed as demoniacal or angelic according to one of the founding "Fathers of Yoga" and a highly regarded Swami as cited here should have been a big enough red flag for me to stop, yet I continued on learning, practicing, and even teaching it to others. What's more, "The Ekagra, the concentrated form of Chitta, is what brings us to Samadhi"[15] and Patanjali's whole purpose of drafting these Yoga Sutras was to "define the technical ways of reaching that state".[16] Samadhi is defined as "a state in which the aspirant is one with the object of his meditation, the Supreme Spirit governing the universe [a cosmotheistic and pantheistic deity], and experiences unutterable peace and joy".[17]

As a believer in Jesus Christ, my soul is completely in despair, even typing out those words now. How could I have yoked myself to this practice knowing the goal was to make myself one with another god, this so-called "Supreme Spirit"? And to attribute it as a goal of reaching some counterfeit to Christ, to achieve the very promises of peace and joy that He gives us, plus so many greater gifts through the Fruits of the Spirit (The Holy Spirit) that we gain when we follow Him. A whole season of repentance took place for me when I finally heeded the conviction, but the good news is, the Gospel is real, and we can be made new through Christ who has already paid the price for these sins, even ones as blatant as this. See even though I had to study all of this to gain my yoga teacher's certificate, and even though I still considered myself a Christian, I fell to the watered-down description that they would give us when anyone asked "Isn't this contrary to religions other than Hinduism, Buddhism, and Jainism", and I chose to listen to the answer, "Well, you can replace the Supreme Spirit" with whatever God you choose... That's the lure, and the devil is a master at manipulation. When I was given that answer, that I could substitute any god or higher power and yoke to it instead, that was the devil operating through those individuals, and what masters they were! They gave me just enough of what I needed to hear to keep me. The devil uses that same tactic in other various aspects of our lives. They go so far in the religious attributes with philosophy, laying the foundations and intentions out so very clearly for us to learn, and just when we get uncomfortable about it, they always provide a scapegoat, a way out that gives us just enough leeway or freedom to convince ourselves that we can still be comfortable, and they keep us hooked. A lot of sin works that way, wouldn't you say?

Iyengar, another modern "father of yoga" who created his own form of yoga known as "Iyengar Yoga" wrote about Patanjali's Yoga Sutras and said, "The uncultured mind fluctuates because of habits of behavior, so he [Patanjali] gives methods of concentrating on the universal spirit of God, or on breath, or on those who have reached liberation through the practice of yoga, or on anything which is congenial to you."[18] You can see so very clearly here where the pantheistic reference of a universal spirit of God is suddenly being swapped for something seemingly so natural and innocent as breathing, to go even further and allude that salvation (or liberation) can come through the practice of yoga (and not Christ alone like the Bible says), and if that's not enough, he just tosses in the final scapegoat statement of "anything congenial to you". I mean, it's hard to argue with that right? Especially when you yourself are trying so hard to take a firm position, it seems there's nothing firm at all to grasp about yoga when you can make it all about whatever you want... Or is there?

The very fact that these types of statements even exist and were written by some of the yogic founders is enough to invalidate the former argument, for there is nothing unsubstantial about taking any other means to connect with our God, outside of God Himself. There is no practice that can yoke you to Him, other than yoking to Him and abiding in Him as we are called to do.

 "Take my yoke upon you and learn from me, for I am gentle and humble in heart, and you will find rest for your souls" (Matthew 11:29, NIV).

"Jesus answered, 'I am the way and the truth and the life. No one comes to the Father except through me.'" (John 14:6, NIV).

THE PROBLEM WITH CHRISTIAN YOGA

Understanding that we are to yoke to Christ alone is fundamental in Christian living. It would also make sense, knowing that Christ is God, that we can not yoke Him to anything. He is God, and we yoke to Him, not the other way around. Trying to yoke Christ to yoga is literally impossible, it is syncretic, and even blasphemous. Yoga is very clearly a pagan practice. We have established enough to know that it was created by vedic priests to yoke to their universal supreme spirit, which is not Christ. We absolutely can not and should stop trying to yoke Christ to anything, let alone a pagan practice.

Idolatry is at the core of yoga, with asanas mimicking false gods and worshiping creation, not The Creator. Perhaps you have heard or done the Suryanamaskar 1 and 2 sequences which are in nearly every single class, and this is a sequence that worships the sun. I'm sure you know about the Warrior 1, 2, and 3 poses, also known as Virabhadrasana, which is named after a demonic warrior, Virabhadra, and the sequence acts out a demonic murder scene from the Bhagavad Gita. If you know all of this, and you think that you can simply change the names of these poses, yet still act them out, and have the Lord look down on you from heaven as your body takes the literal shape of a demon beheading people at a wedding like the story goes, then you are lying to yourself. It does not matter what the intention of your heart is, for the Bible says our hearts are evil and can not be trusted. If you are calling it yoga, and you are doing the poses, and your body is showing up mimicking false gods, demons, and worshiping idols, then surely you must know that is what the Lord sees too.

WHAT'S REALLY WRONG WITH JUST DOING THE POSES?

When our bodies assume positions that were intentionally created by pagans to mimic, yoke, and worship their false gods or facets of creation, then we see these once seemingly just harmless yoga poses as much more. We see them for what they are, a blatant invitation for whatever spirit (demon) attached to these poses to enter into our lives and wreak havoc. This is spiritual warfare 101. The devil is a legalist, and when he gains a right of passage into our life, he takes all the ground he can. Ephesians 4:27 says, "and do not give the devil a foothold". Would participating in an ancient pagan spiritual worship practice be a foothold? Yes!

Have you ever stopped to wonder why, out of all the other forms of "exercise", they are never considered to be a practice (outside of yoga)? One does not say, "I have a solid aerobics practice", or "I practice weightlifting". No, this is not the same because yoga is not the same as regular exercise or fitness. It is very much a practice, and what is a practice for? A practice is intended to be perfected, to be done so often and so comprehensively that it can be done automatically, like a routine, without having to think. Maybe a doctor or surgeon is a good reference here, and they are said to practice medicine, so that when the time comes to act, they do not have to think, they can simply treat the patient. They are not looking at books of "how to operate" when the patient is on the surgery table, one would hope! A practice seeps into the depths of your mind and body, and uniquely of yoga, also your soul. 1 John 3:8-10 says, "Whoever makes a practice of sinning is of the devil, for the devil has been sinning from the beginning. The reason the Son of God appeared was to destroy the works of the devil. No one born of God makes a practice of sinning, for God's seed abides in him, and he cannot keep on sinning because he has been born of God. By this it is evident who are the children of God, and who are the children of the devil: whoever does not practice righteousness is not of God, nor is the one who does not love his brother." I find this verse and the fact that yoga is not just an act, it is not just something that you can casually dabble in, its intent and those of the demonic spirits operating behind it are to ensnare you into making a practice of it, and it is sin. Moreso, it is one of the major sins that we see provokes God to a jealous anger, the worship of other gods.

There are so many truly wonderful modes of fitness and exercise available that do not have this ancient pagan roots that they are yoking you to. When the practice as a whole means "to yoke", and it is a pagan spiritual practice with every aspect intentionally created to unite, worship, or mimic us to things that are NOT Jesus Christ, then we as Christians must pause and ask ourselves, "Is this really worth it?" The Lord created us, as His New Creations, to be His vessels on earth. Yoga talks about our bodies becoming temples, but unto what? Surely, after reading all of this, you can see that these two temples, the one where we become temples of the Holy Spirit as Beliver's, and the one where we are yoking in union to pagan entities, are NOT one in the same. There are not many paths that lead to God as the New Age and yoga will tell you. There is Only One.

Mark 12:30-31 tells us, "Love the Lord your God with all your heart and with all your soul and with all your mind and with all your strength.The second is this: 'Love your neighbor as yourself.'There is no commandment greater than these." Is it loving to let your neighbor perish for lack of knowledge on topics so very deceptive as this? Most people truly do not know the truth about yoga, because they have been blinded by either false teachers, or those who simply lack the understanding and have not been curious enough to do the research to learn. My prayer is that this will spare my fellow brothers and sisters in Christ from suffering the repercussions and consequences of engaging in a pagan spiritual practice that I had to incur. The Lord is just, and He is good, and He forgives us of our sins, but that does not mean that we will not still suffer the consequences of our actions.

May The Lord grant you His peace, His wisdom, and His grace on this matter.

In His love,

Michal Russo

BIBLIOGRAPHY

Allard, S. (2020, September 23). *Who Was Patanjali and What Are The Yoga Sutras?* Hindu American Foundation. https://www.hinduamerican.org/blog/who-was-patanjali-and-what-are-the-yoga-sutras

Geno, R. (2021, June 14). The meaning of namaste. *Yoga Journal.* https://www.yogajournal.com/practice/beginners/the-meaning-of-namaste/

Bugnini, A. (1953). Documenta pontificia ad instaurationem liturgicam spectantia. *Roma: Edizioni Liturgiche, 1953-1959.*, 6(9), 18.

Iyengar, B. K. S. (1989). *The Tree of Yoga: Yoga*

vṛkṣa. Shambhala Publications.

Lark, L. (2008). *1,001 pearls of yoga wisdom: Take your practice beyond the mat* (p. 267). Chronicle Books.

Liturgical languages. (n.d.). Encyclopedia.Com. Retrieved February 7, 2022, from https://www.encyclopedia.com/religion/encyclopedias-almanacs-transcripts-and-maps/liturgical-languages

Vivekananda, S. (2021). *Patanjali Yoga Sutras.* Sristhi Publishers & Distributors.

---

[1] Geno, R. (2021, June 14). The meaning of namaste. *Yoga Journal.* https://www.yogajournal.com/practice/beginners/the-meaning-of-namaste/

[2] Ibid.

[3] Lark, L. (2008). *1,001 pearls of yoga wisdom: Take your practice beyond the mat* (p. 267). Chronicle Books.

[4] *Liturgical languages.* (n.d.). Encyclopedia.Com. Retrieved February 7, 2022, from https://www.encyclopedia.com/

religion/encyclopedias-almanacs-transcripts-and-maps/
liturgical-languages

[5] Ibid.

[6] Allard, S. (2020, September 23). *Who Was Patanjali and What Are The Yoga Sutras?* Hindu American Foundation. https://www.hinduamerican.org/blog/who-was-patanjali-and-what-are-the-yoga-sutras

[7] Ibid.

[8] Vivekananda, S. (2021). *Patanjali Yoga Sutras*. Sristhi Publishers & Distributors.

[9] Ibid., 9

[10] Ibid., 13

[11] Idid.

[12] Ibid.

[13] Ibid.

[14] Ibid.

[15] Ibid.

[16] Iyengar, B. K. S. (1989). *The Tree of Yoga: Yoga vṛkṣa*. Shambhala Publications., 119.

[17] Ibid., 179

[18] Iyengar, B. K. S. (1989). *The Tree of Yoga: Yoga vṛkṣa*. Shambhala Publications., 119-120.

ABOUT THE AUTHOR

Michal Russo

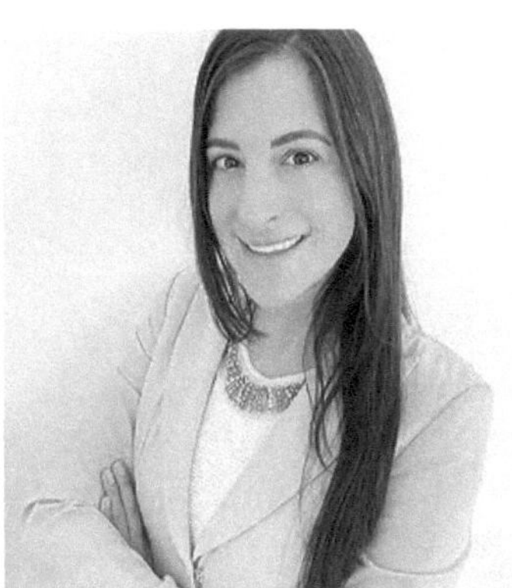

Michal Russo is a wife, mother, author, speaker, and founder of fitness ministry "WorshipFlow", a Christian faith-based alternative to yoga. As a former yoga instructor and New Age practitioner, Michal is passionate about sharing her powerful reformation story of inner healing, health, and wellness through a life lived for Christ. Journey with her through spiritually sound practices that can be implemented into your life today.

BOOKS BY THIS AUTHOR

7 Steps To Realign Body, Soul, Spirit

This wasn't, and isn't, an easy assignment, answering the call by God to share my story of crashing and burning that led me to a total realignment of body, soul, and spirit in Faith by Grace. The further I pursued the Faith, the block came. Like a physical & spiritual stop sign that no longer allowed me to continue practicing yoga let alone teach it. Like any ritual that you practice so often it becomes automatic, yoga had become my whole world. From my career, to yogi friends, to my actual identity; it involved my entire body and soul, and unknowingly my spirit too. I longed for that time where I felt like I was flowing, and like I was aligned, often how I had convinced myself I felt during yoga. I knew I needed a complete restoration, from the inside-out, and that it had to involve more than just my body and soul now, because my spirit had finally been awakened to what it had been yoking to, and it was not Christ. I will go into more depth on the truth about yoga later in this book, as it took me certain steps that I had to reach first to accept this knowledge and I realize that it may also be that way for you too. I want to be clear and intentional about my faith, and His sweet mercy and grace. I knew I wanted to help others by sharing my experience so that they could find restoration and realignment in faith, by grace.